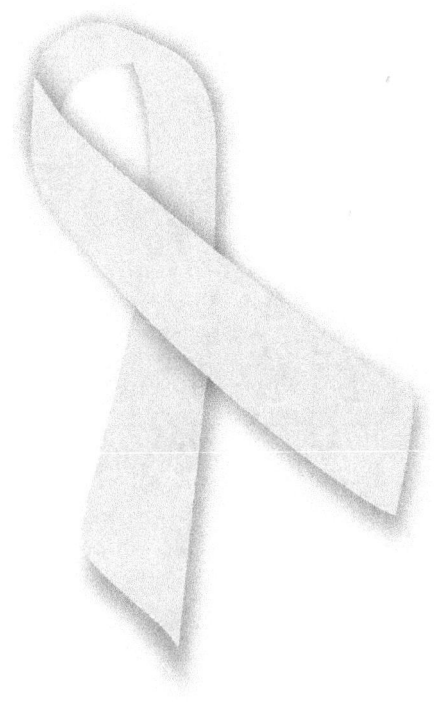

Unraveling The Mystery: Understanding

# Lyme Disease

Migdalia Mugan

# Table of contents

# Introduction

Lyme disease is a tick-borne illness caused by the bacterium Borrelia burgdorferi. It is the most commonly reported vector-borne disease in the United States and Europe. The disease is named after the town of Lyme, Connecticut, where it was first identified in 1975. Transmission of Lyme disease occurs primarily through the bite of infected black-legged ticks, commonly known as deer ticks. These ticks become infected after feeding on infected animals, such as deer or mice. Humans can then contract the disease when bitten by an infected tick.

The symptoms of Lyme disease can vary and typically develop in three stages:

### Early localized stage

Within a few days to weeks after a tick bite, an expanding red rash called erythema migrans (EM) may appear at the site of the tick bite. The rash is often circular and has a bull's-eye appearance, but it can also be solid red. Other symptoms during this stage may include fatigue, fever, headache, muscle and joint aches, and swollen lymph nodes.

## Early disseminated stage

If left untreated, the infection can spread throughout the body, leading to more widespread symptoms. These may include additional EM rashes in different areas, flu-like symptoms (fever, chills, fatigue), headache, neck stiffness, muscle and joint aches, and swollen lymph nodes. In some cases, neurological symptoms such as facial paralysis, dizziness, and cognitive difficulties can occur.

## Late persistent stage

If Lyme disease is still untreated, it can progress to the late stage, which may develop months or even years after the initial infection. Symptoms may include severe fatigue, joint pain and swelling (particularly in the knees), memory problems, difficulty concentrating, and sleep disturbances. Some individuals may experience ongoing neurological issues, such as tingling or numbness in the hands or feet. Diagnosing Lyme disease can be challenging as the symptoms can mimic other conditions, and laboratory tests may yield false negatives in the early stages. Doctors typically consider symptoms, medical history, and possible exposure to infected ticks when making a diagnosis.

Early treatment with appropriate antibiotics, such as doxycycline, amoxicillin, or cefuroxime, is crucial to prevent the progression of Lyme disease. In most cases, prompt treatment can lead to a complete recovery. However, if the disease is not detected and treated early, it can cause long-term complications affecting the joints, heart, and nervous system.

Preventing Lyme disease involves taking precautions when spending time in areas where ticks are common, such as wooded or grassy areas. These precautions include wearing protective clothing, using insect repellents containing DEET, conducting regular tick checks, and promptly removing ticks from the body.

In conclusion, Lyme disease is a tick-borne illness caused by the bacterium Borrelia burgdorferi. It can lead to a range of symptoms affecting multiple body systems. Early diagnosis and treatment are essential to prevent complications and ensure a full recovery. Taking preventive measures to avoid tick bites is crucial for reducing the risk of contracting the disease.

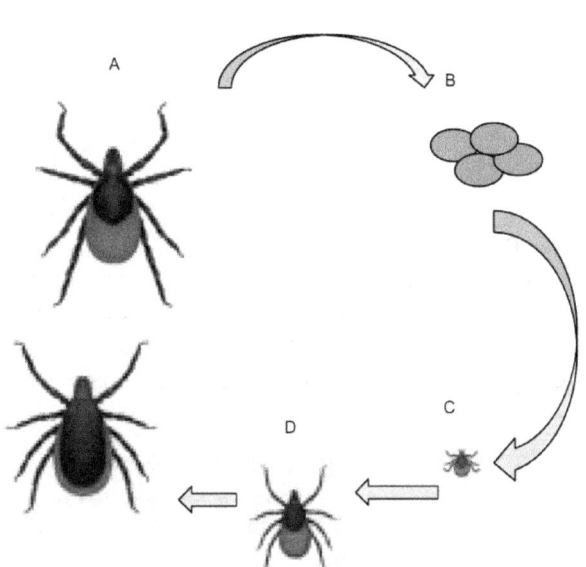

**Chapter 1**: Introduction to Lyme Disease: History, Prevalence, and Impact

## 1.1 History of Lyme Disease

The history of Lyme disease is a fascinating tale of discovery and scientific investigation. In the early 1970s, a group of concerned mothers in Lyme, Connecticut, noticed a cluster of children experiencing unusual symptoms, including joint pain, fatigue, and a distinct circular rash. This caught the attention of researchers, leading to investigations by Dr. Allen Steere and his team.

Through rigorous study and collaboration, it was discovered that the disease, initially named "Lyme arthritis," was associated with tick bites. The connection between the deer tick (Ixodes scapularis) and the transmission of the disease was established.

Further research led to the identification of the bacterium responsible for the illness, named Borrelia burgdorferi, after Dr. Willy Burgdorfer, who played a key role in its isolation.

## 1.2 Global Prevalence of Lyme Disease

Lyme disease is not limited to the town of Lyme, Connecticut. It has become a global health concern. Regions where Lyme disease is endemic include parts of North America, particularly the northeastern and upper midwestern United States, as well as areas of Europe, Asia, and Australia.

The prevalence of Lyme disease varies across these regions. In some areas, such as the northeastern United States, it is a significant public health issue, with thousands of reported cases each year.

In Europe, countries like Germany and Austria also experience a high incidence of Lyme disease. Additionally, there are emerging areas of concern where the disease is being recognized more frequently, highlighting the need for increased awareness and surveillance.

## 1.3 Impact of Lyme Disease

Lyme disease can have a profound impact on affected individuals, communities, and public health. The physical symptoms of Lyme disease, such as joint pain, muscle aches, and fatigue, can be debilitating, affecting daily activities and reducing quality of life.

Untreated or undiagnosed cases can lead to more severe complications, including neurological disorders, heart problems, and long-term joint damage.

The emotional toll of Lyme disease should not be underestimated. Chronic symptoms and the challenges in diagnosis and treatment can lead to frustration, anxiety, and depression.

Furthermore, the socioeconomic impact of Lyme disease is significant. The costs associated with medical care, missed workdays, and reduced productivity can strain individuals, families, and healthcare systems.

## 1.4 Public Awareness and Advocacy

Raising public awareness and promoting advocacy for Lyme disease are crucial endeavors. Patient advocacy groups, healthcare organizations, and government agencies play an essential role in educating the public about prevention, early recognition, and appropriate treatment. Efforts are made to dispel misconceptions surrounding the disease, address controversies related to chronic Lyme disease, and ensure accurate information is readily available.

Improving education for healthcare providers is also vital. Enhancing their knowledge about Lyme disease symptoms, diagnostic methods, and treatment options can lead to earlier detection and more effective management. Additionally, fostering a supportive environment for individuals living with Lyme disease, providing resources, and encouraging community engagement are vital aspects of advocacy.

## 1.5 Current Research and Areas of Study

Research on Lyme disease continues to evolve, leading to advancements in diagnosis, treatment, and prevention strategies. Scientists are studying tick biology, the complex interactions between Borrelia burgdorferi and the human immune system, and the development of more accurate diagnostic tools.

New diagnostic techniques, such as improved serological tests and molecular assays, are being developed to enhance early detection and reduce false negatives. Vaccine research, both for humans and potentially for animals, is ongoing to prevent Lyme disease transmission. Additionally, novel prevention strategies, including the development of tick-control methods and public health interventions, are areas of active investigation.

Collaboration between academia, healthcare professionals, and public health agencies is vital to address the challenges posed by Lyme disease effectively. These collaborative efforts aim to improve diagnostics, refine treatment protocols, enhance public awareness, and ultimately reduce the burden of Lyme disease on individuals and communities.

**Chapter 2:** The Tick and the Bacterium:
Understanding Borrelia burgdorferi


2.1 Tick Vectors and Their Life Cycle

This section delves into the world of tick vectors, specifically the black-legged ticks (Ixodes scapularis and Ixodes pacificus) commonly associated with Lyme disease transmission. It discusses the life cycle of ticks, including the egg, larva, nymph, and adult stages

. The chapter explains how ticks acquire the bacterium Borrelia burgdorferi by feeding on infected reservoir hosts, such as mice, birds, or deer, during different stages of their life cycle.

## 2.2 Borrelia burgdorferi: The Causative Agent

This section focuses on the bacterium Borrelia burgdorferi, the causative agent of Lyme disease. It explores the structure and characteristics of Borrelia burgdorferi, such as its spiral shape and unique ability to evade the immune system. The chapter delves into the genetic diversity of Borrelia burgdorferi strains and how this variation contributes to differences in disease presentation and severity.

## 2.3 Transmission of Borrelia burgdorferi

The transmission process of Borrelia burgdorferi from infected ticks to humans is a key aspect of understanding Lyme disease. This section explains how ticks become infected with Borrelia burgdorferi by feeding on infected reservoir hosts. It discusses the complex interactions that occur during tick feeding, including the migration of the bacterium from the tick's midgut to its salivary glands. The chapter also highlights the role of tick saliva in modulating the host immune response and facilitating the transmission of the bacterium.

2.4 Pathogenesis of Lyme Disease

Understanding the pathogenesis of Lyme disease is crucial for comprehending the diverse symptoms and clinical manifestations. This section explores how Borrelia burgdorferi interacts with the human body upon infection. It discusses the bacterium's ability to invade various tissues, including the skin, joints, heart, and nervous system. The chapter also delves into the immune response triggered by Borrelia burgdorferi, including both innate and adaptive immunity, and how the bacterium can evade or manipulate these responses.

2.5 Tick Bite Avoidance and Personal Protection

To prevent Lyme disease, it is important to take measures to avoid tick bites. This section provides practical information on tick bite prevention and personal protection strategies. It covers topics such as wearing protective clothing, using insect repellents, conducting regular tick checks, and implementing environmental modifications to reduce tick habitat. The chapter emphasizes the importance of these prevention measures in reducing the risk of tick bites and subsequent Lyme disease                         transmission.

## Transmission

The Lyme disease bacteria causing human infection in the United States, Borrelia burgdorferi and, rarely, B. mayonii, are spread to people through the bites of infected ticks.

Borrelia burgdorferi is spread primarily by the blacklegged tick (deer tick, Ixodes scapularis) in the northeastern, mid-Atlantic, and north- central United States, and by the western black legged tick (I.pacificus) in the Pacific Coast states. Borrelia mayonii is rarely found in ticks and has only been detected in blacklegged ticks in the north-central United States.

Blacklegged ticks have a 2-3 year life cycle. During this time, they go through four life stages: egg, larva, nymph and adult. After the egg hatches, the larva and nymph each must take a blood meal to develop to the next life stage, and the female needs blood to produce eggs.

. Larva and nymphal ticks can become infected with Lyme disease bacteria when feeding on an infected wildlife host, usually a rodent. The bacteria are passed along to the next life stage. Nymphs or adult females can then spread the bacteria during their next blood meal.

. Female ticks infected with Lyme disease bacteria do not pass them to their offspring.

. Deer are important sources of blood for ticks and are important to tick survival and movement to new areas. However, deer are not infected with the Lyme disease bacteria and do not infect ticks.

In most cases, a tick must be attacked for 36 to 48 hours or more before the Lyme disease bacterium can be transmitted. If you remove a tick quickly (within 24 hours), you can greatly reduce your chances of getting Lyme disease.

April through July, nymphs are actively questing for hosts in the environment, and in early spring and fall seasons, adults are most active.

Nymphal ticks pose a particularly high risk due to their abundance and small size ( about the size of a poppy seed), which makes them difficult to spot.

In fact, lyme disease patients are often not aware of a tick bite before getting sick.

Adult female ticks also can transmit the bacteria but because of their larger size are more likely to be noticed and removed from people before transmission of the bacteria can occur.

# Life Cycle of the *Ixodes scapularis* Tick

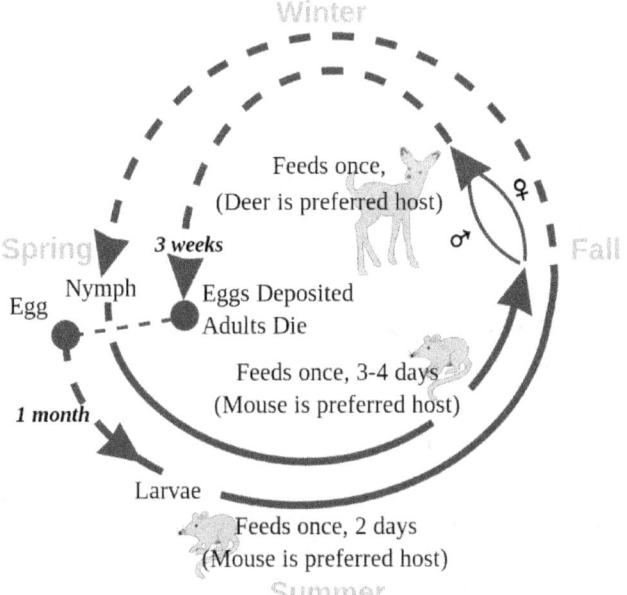

Winter

Feeds once,
(Deer is preferred host)

Spring

3 weeks

Egg

Nymph

Eggs Deposited
Adults Die

Feeds once, 3-4 days
(Mouse is preferred host)

Fall

1 month

Larvae

Feeds once, 2 days
(Mouse is preferred host)

Summer

## Prevention of Tick bites

### Before going Outdoors

. Know where to expect ticks. Ticks live in grassy, bushy, or wooded areas, or even on animals. Spending time outside walking your dog, camping , gardening or hunting could bring you in close contact with ticks. Many people get ticks in their own yard.

. Treat clothing and gear with products containing 0.5% permethrin. Permethrin can be used to treat boots, clothing and camping gear and remain protective through several washings.

. Use Environmental Protection Agency (EPA)-registered insect repellents containing DEET, picaridin, IR3535,oil of lemon eucalyptus (OLE), para menthane-diol (PMD), or 2-undecanone.

. Avoid contact with ticks- Avoid wooded and bushy areas with high grass and leaf litter and walk in the center of trails.

After coming indoors

Check your clothing for ticks. Ticks may be carried into the house on clothing. Any ticks that are found should be removed. Tumble dry clothes in a dryer on high heat for 10 minutes to kill it.

Examine gear and pets. Ticks can ride into the home on clothing and pets, then attach to a person later, so carefully examine pets coats and backpacks.

Shower soon after being outdoors.
 Showering within two hours of coming indoors has been shown to reduce your risk of getting Lyme disease and may be effective in reducing the risk of other tick borne diseases. Showering may help wash off unattached ticks and it's a good opportunity to do a tick check.

Check your body for ticks after being outdoors. Conduct a full body check upon return form potentially ick-infected areas, including your own backyard.

Use a hand-held mirror or full-length mirror to view all parts of your body.

. Under the arms

. In and around the ears

. Inside belly button

. Back of knees

. In and around the hair

. Between the legs

. Around the waist

. In your scalp

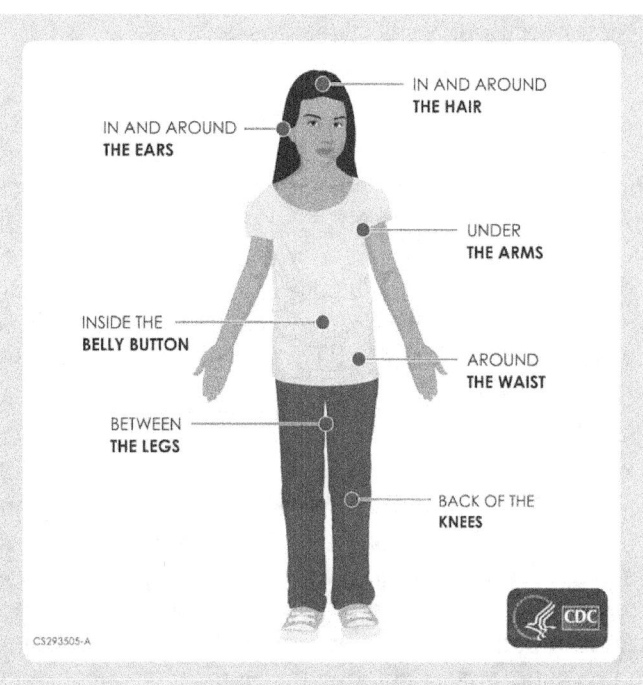

IN AND AROUND
**THE HAIR**

IN AND AROUND
**THE EARS**

UNDER
**THE ARMS**

INSIDE THE
**BELLY BUTTON**

AROUND
**THE WAIST**

BETWEEN
**THE LEGS**

BACK OF THE
**KNEES**

CS293505-A

## Post- treatment Lyme disease syndrome

Lyme disease is caused by infection with the bacterium Borrelia burgdorferi. Although most cases can be cured with a 2-4 weeks course of oral antibiotics, patients can sometimes have symptoms of pain, fatigue or difficulty thinking that last for more than 6 months after they finish treatment. This condition is called Post-Treatment Lyme Disease Syndrome (PTLDS).

Many experts believe that PTLDS may be caused due the bacteria Borrelia burgdorferi triggering an "auto-immune" response causing  symptoms that last well after the infection itself is gone. Auto-immune responses are known to occur following other infections, including  campylobacter (Guillain-barre syndrome),  chlamydia (reactive arthritis), and strep throat (rheumatic heart disease).

Other experts believe that PTLDS results  from a persistent but difficult to detect infection. Finally, others think the symptoms of PTLDS are due to other causes unrelated to the patient's Borrelia burgdorferi                                        infection.

**Chapter 3**: Signs and Symptoms: Recognizing Lyme Disease


3.1 Early Localized Stage

This section focuses on the signs and symptoms that are typically observed during the early localized stage of Lyme disease. It explores the primary hallmark of this stage: the appearance of erythema migrans (EM) rash.

The chapter explains the characteristics of the EM rash, including its circular or oval shape, redness, and potential for a bull's-eye appearance. It also emphasizes that not all EM rashes have a classic appearance and that they can vary in size and presentation.

Additionally, the section discusses other common symptoms that may accompany the EM rash during the early localized stage. These may include fatigue, fever, headache, muscle and joint aches, and swollen lymph nodes.

The chapter highlights the importance of recognizing these symptoms in conjunction with the presence of an EM rash for early diagnosis and treatment.

## 3.2 Early Disseminated Stage

In this section, the chapter explores the signs and symptoms that may manifest during the early disseminated stage of Lyme disease. It explains that if left untreated, the infection can spread beyond the site of the tick bite and affect multiple body systems.

The section discusses the occurrence of multiple EM rashes in different areas of the body as a characteristic feature of the early disseminated stage.

It highlights the importance of distinguishing these rashes from other skin conditions. Furthermore, the chapter delves into additional symptoms that may be present during this stage, such as flu-like symptoms (fever, chills, fatigue), headache, neck stiffness, muscle and joint aches, and swollen lymph nodes.

It also discusses the possibility of neurological symptoms, including facial paralysis, dizziness, and cognitive difficulties.

## 3.3 Late Persistent Stage

This section focuses on the signs and symptoms that may arise during the late persistent stage of Lyme disease. It explains that this stage can occur months or even years after the initial infection, particularly if Lyme disease remains untreated.

The chapter explores the symptoms commonly observed during the late persistent stage, which may vary from person to person. It discusses the presence of severe fatigue, often referred to as "Lyme fatigue," which can be debilitating and impact daily functioning.

It also delves into the prevalence of joint pain and swelling, particularly in the knees, as a characteristic manifestation of late-stage Lyme disease.

Additionally, the section explores other symptoms that may be present, such as memory problems, difficulty concentrating, sleep disturbances, and mood changes. It may touch upon the potential for ongoing neurological issues, such as tingling or numbness in the hands or feet.

## 3.4 Diagnostic Challenges and Considerations

This section addresses the challenges and considerations related to diagnosing Lyme disease. It discusses the limitations of diagnostic tests, including the potential for false negatives, particularly during the early stages of the disease. The chapter explores the importance of considering clinical symptoms, medical history, and potential exposure to infected ticks when making a diagnosis.

Furthermore, the section explores the role of serological tests, such as enzyme immunoassays (EIAs) and Western blot tests, in confirming a diagnosis of Lyme disease. It discusses the interpretation of test results and the challenges associated with serological testing, including the possibility of false positives and the need for clinical correlation.

The chapter also highlights the importance of healthcare providers being knowledgeable about the diagnostic guidelines and recommendations specific to their region. It emphasizes the significance of considering Lyme disease as a potential diagnosis in areas where the disease is endemic, even in the absence of a classic EM rash.

The symptoms of Lyme Disease

Stage I
Early symptoms of Lyme disease usually happen within 3 to 30 days after a tick bite. Thai stage of disease has a limited set of symptoms. This is called early localized disease.

A rash is a common sign of Lyme disease. But it does not always happen. The rash is usually a single circle that slowly spreads from the site of the tick bite. It may become clear in the center and look like a target or bull's eye.  The rash often feels warm to the touch, but it's usually not painful or itchy.

Other stage 1 symptoms include:
. Fever
. Headaches
. Extreme tiredness
. Joint stiffness
. Muscle aches and pains
. Swollen lymph nodes.

## Stage II

Without treatment, lyme disease can get worse. The symptoms often show up within 3 to 10 weeks after a  tick bite. Stage II is often more serious and widespread. It's called early disseminated disease.

Stage II may include the stage I symptoms  and the following:

. Many rashes on other parts of the body.

.Neck pain or stiffness.

. Muscle weakness on one or both sides of the face.

. Immune-system activity in heart tissue that causes irregular heartbeats.

. Pain that starts from the back and hips and spreads to the legs.

. Painful swelling in tissues of the eye or eyelid.

. Immune-system activity in eye nerves that causes pain or vision loss.

## Stage III

In the third stage, you may have symptoms from the earlier stages and other symptoms. The stage is called late disseminated disease.

In the United States, the most common condition of this stage is arthritis in large joints, particularly in the knees. Pain , swelling or stiffness may last for a long time. Or the symptoms may come and go. Stage III symptoms usually begin 2 to 12 months after a tick bite.

The type of Lyme disease common in Europe can cause a skin condition called acrodermatitis chronic atrophicans. The skin on the back of the hands and tops of the feet get discolored and swell. It also may show up over the elbows and knees. More- serious cases may cause damage to the tissues or joints.

## When to see a doctor

Most people who get Lyme disease don't recall getting a tick bite. And many symptoms of Lyme disease relate to other conditions. See your doctor if you have Lyme disease symptoms. A prompt diagnosis and proper treatment can improve outcomes.

**Chapter 4**: Diagnostic Methods and Challenges

4.1 Serological Testing for Lyme Disease

This section focuses on the serological testing methods used for diagnosing Lyme disease. It explains the two-step approach recommended by most guidelines: an initial enzyme immunoassay (EIA) followed by a confirmatory Western blot test.

The chapter discusses the rationale behind this two-step process and the specific antibodies targeted by these tests.

Furthermore, the section explores the limitations and challenges associated with serological testing for Lyme disease. It highlights the potential for false-negative results, particularly in the early stages of the disease when antibody levels may not be detectable.

The chapter explains that serological testing is most reliable in later stages when antibody production is more pronounced.

The chapter also addresses the issue of false-positive results in serological testing. It discusses the possibility of cross-reactivity with antibodies generated against other pathogens, such as the bacteria that cause syphilis or certain viral infections.

The section emphasizes the importance of clinical correlation and considering the patient's symptoms and exposure history when interpreting serological test results.

## 4.2 Polymerase Chain Reaction (PCR) Testing

This section delves into the role of polymerase chain reaction (PCR) testing in diagnosing Lyme disease.

It explains that PCR testing involves detecting the genetic material (DNA) of Borrelia burgdorferi in a patient's blood, joint fluid, or tissue samples.

The chapter discusses the potential advantages of PCR testing, such as its ability to detect the presence of the bacterium even in the early stages of                              the                              disease.

However, the section also addresses the limitations of PCR testing for Lyme disease.

It explains that PCR testing may yield false-negative results if the bacterium is not present in sufficient quantities or if the samples are not collected at the appropriate time.

The chapter emphasizes that PCR testing is most useful when combined with clinical evaluation and other diagnostic methods.

## 4.3 Clinical Assessment and Considerations

This section explores the importance of clinical assessment and considerations in diagnosing Lyme disease.

It highlights the significance of evaluating a patient's medical history, physical examination findings, and exposure to tick-infested areas.

The chapter discusses the role of healthcare providers in conducting a thorough clinical evaluation and considering Lyme disease as a potential diagnosis.

Furthermore, the section explores the challenges in diagnosing Lyme disease based solely on clinical presentation.

It discusses the wide range of symptoms and the potential overlap with other conditions, making diagnosis based on symptoms alone difficult.

The chapter emphasizes the importance of integrating clinical assessment with laboratory testing for accurate diagnosis.

### 4.4 Challenges in Diagnosis and Future Directions

This section addresses the challenges in diagnosing Lyme disease and highlights areas for future research and improvement.

It discusses the need for more accurate and reliable diagnostic tests, particularly for early-stage Lyme disease where antibody levels may be low.

The chapter explores ongoing research efforts to develop new diagnostic tools, such as improved serological assays or point-of-care tests for rapid diagnosis.

**The Most common symptoms of Lyme disease**

. Erythema migran (EM) rash- A bulls-eye rash that appears at the site of the tick bite, usually within 3-30 days after the tick bite. The rash can expand to become a large red area and may or may not be itchy or painful.

. Flu-like symptoms: fever, chills, fatigue, headaches , muscle and joint aches, and swollen lymph nodes.

. Neurological symptoms: Difficulty concentrating, memory problems and headaches. Some people may also experience facial palsy, which is temporary weakness or drooping of the facial muscles.

. Cardiovascular symptoms- irregular heartbeats, or chest pain.

. Arthritis: Joint pain and swelling , especially in the knees.

. Bell's palsy- It's a sudden weakness or paralysis of the muscles on one side of the face.

. Irritable bowel syndrome

.                         Sleep                  disturbances

**Testing for Lyme disease**

. Most Lyme disease tests are designed to detect antibodies made by the body in response to infection.

. Antibodies can take several weeks to develop, so patients may test negative if infected only recently.

. Antibodies normally persist in the blood for months or even years after  the infection is gone; therefore,  the test cannot be used to determine cure.

. Some tests give results for two types of antibody, IgM and IgG. Positive IgM results should be disregarded if the patient has been ill for more than 30                                                        days.

## Laboratory testing

The CDC recommends a two step testing process for Lyme disease. Both tests are required and can be done using the same blood sample.

If this first step is negative, no further testing is required. If the first test is positive or indeterminate (equivocal), the second step should be performed.

The overall result is positive only when the first step is positive (or equivocal) and the second test is positive (or for some tests equivocal).

One of these tests is called the ELISA test and you will often have a second test called the Western blot                                                    test.

**Chapter 5**: Treatment Approaches: Antibiotics and Beyond

5.1 Antibiotic Treatment for Lyme Disease

This section focuses on the primary treatment approach for Lyme disease: antibiotic therapy. It discusses the commonly prescribed antibiotics, such as doxycycline, amoxicillin, and cefuroxime, and their effectiveness in combating Borrelia burgdorferi infection. The chapter explores the rationale behind selecting specific antibiotics based on the stage of the disease and patient-specific factors, such as age, pregnancy, and allergies.

Furthermore, the section provides guidance on the duration of antibiotic treatment. It discusses the recommended treatment durations for different stages of Lyme disease, considering factors such as the extent of infection, the presence of symptoms, and the individual's response to treatment. The chapter emphasizes the importance of completing the full course of antibiotics as prescribed to ensure the eradication of the bacterium and prevent the development of complications.

The standard treatment for Lyme disease involves the use of antibiotics. Here are the main treatments used for Lyme disease:

Antibiotics:

- **Doxycycline:**This is the preferred antibiotic for most adults and children over 8 years old. It is effective against early-stage Lyme disease and can be administered orally.
- **Amoxicillin:** This is the first-line treatment for pregnant women and young children under 8 years old. It is also effective against early-stage Lyme disease and is given orally.
- **Cefuroxime:** This antibiotic is used as an alternative to doxycycline or amoxicillin for adults and children who cannot tolerate those drugs or if there are other medical considerations. It is also given orally.

Intravenous Antibiotics:

⊠ **Ceftriaxone:**

In cases where the infection has spread to the central nervous system or when oral antibiotics have not effectively treated the disease, intravenous antibiotics may be prescribed. Ceftriaxone is commonly used for this purpose.

Duration of Treatment:
- The duration of treatment typically depends on the stage of Lyme disease, the severity of symptoms, and the individual's response to antibiotics. Early-stage Lyme disease is often treated with a 2-4 week course of antibiotics, while more advanced or complicated cases may require longer treatment.

Follow-up:
- After completing the antibiotic course, patients should have regular follow-up appointments with their healthcare provider to monitor their progress and ensure that the infection has been fully treated.

Pain Relief:
- For patients with persistent joint or muscle pain, over-the-counter pain relievers like acetaminophen or ibuprofen can be used to manage discomfort.

It's essential to remember that early diagnosis and prompt treatment are crucial for successful recovery from Lyme disease. If you suspect you may have been exposed to ticks or are experiencing symptoms consistent with Lyme disease (e.g., fever, headache, fatigue, joint pain, and a characteristic "bull's-eye" rash), seek medical attention immediately.

As always, please consult a healthcare professional for personalized advice and treatment recommendations for Lyme disease or any other medical condition.

## The Interdisciplinary Team

The treatment of Lyme disease often involves an interdisciplinary approach, with various healthcare professionals working together to provide comprehensive care. The interdisciplinary team aims to address the diverse aspects of Lyme disease, including diagnosis, treatment, symptom management, and long-term support. The following are some of the key members of the interdisciplinary team involved in the treatment of Lyme disease:

**Primary Care Physician:**

The primary care physician (PCP) is usually the first point of contact for patients with suspected Lyme disease. They conduct initial evaluations, order tests for diagnosis, and may prescribe antibiotics or refer the patient to a specialist if necessary.

**Infectious Disease Specialists:**

An infectious disease specialist is a medical doctor with expertise in diagnosing and treating infection diseases like Lyme disease. They often lead the treatment plan for more complex or advanced cases.

**Rheumatologist:**

For patients experiencing persistent joint pain and inflammation, a rheumatologist may be involved in managing arthritis-like symptoms associated with late-stage or chronic Lyme disease.

**Neurologist:**

In cases where Lyme disease affects the nervous system, a neurologist may be consulted to manage neurological symptoms and complications.

**Pain Management Specialist:**

Some patients with Lyme disease may require additional pain management strategies to address persistent pain. A pain management specialist can provide expertise in managing pain and improving the patient's quality of life.

**Physical Therapist:**

Physical therapists can play a crucial role in helping patients regain strength, mobility, and function during the recovery process. They can develop tailored exercise programs and therapeutic techniques to address specific physical limitations caused by the disease.

**Occupational Therapist:**

Occupational therapists help patients improve their ability to perform daily tasks and activities while adapting to any functional limitations caused by Lyme disease.

**Mental Health Professionals:**

Lyme disease can have significant psychological effects on patients, particularly when symptoms are prolonged or severe. Mental health professionals, such as psychologists or psychiatrists, can provide counseling and support to address anxiety, depression, and other emotional challenges.

**Nurse:**

Nurses play a critical role in patient education, monitoring treatment progress, and providing ongoing care and support.

**Laboratory Specialists:**

Medical laboratory professionals are involved in conducting tests to diagnose Lyme disease and monitor treatment effectiveness.

**Social Worker or Case Manager:**

Social workers or case managers can help coordinate care and provide assistance with accessing resources and support services.

**Patient and Family:**

The patient and their family play an essential role in the treatment team. Their active participation in treatment decisions and adherence to the prescribed treatment plan are crucial for successful outcomes.

Effective communication and collaboration among these interdisciplinary team members are vital for providing comprehensive and coordinated care to individuals with Lyme disease. This approach ensures that all aspects of the disease are addressed, leading to better patient outcomes and quality of life.

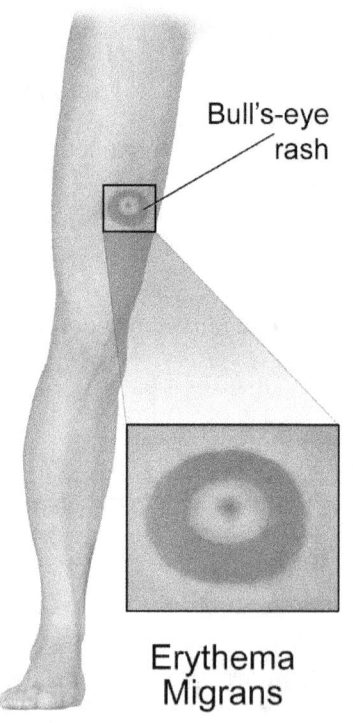

Bull's-eye rash

Erythema Migrans

5.2 Management of Persistent or Chronic Lyme Disease

This section addresses the management of persistent or chronic Lyme disease, which refers to cases where symptoms persist or recur despite appropriate antibiotic treatment.

The chapter discusses the challenges in managing these cases and the lack of consensus on optimal treatment approaches.

The section explores various strategies and considerations for managing persistent or chronic Lyme disease symptoms. It may touch upon the use of extended antibiotic therapy, such as intravenous (IV) antibiotics, in specific cases where there is evidence of ongoing infection or severe symptoms.

The chapter also discusses the importance of a multidisciplinary approach, involving specialists such as rheumatologists, neurologists, and pain management experts, to address specific symptoms and provide comprehensive care.

Furthermore, the section explores non-antibiotic treatment options for managing persistent or chronic symptoms.

It may discuss the potential role of anti-inflammatory medications, pain management strategies, physical therapy, and complementary therapies, such as acupuncture or herbal remedies.

The chapter emphasizes the need for individualized treatment plans tailored to each patient's specific symptoms and needs.

## 5.3 Emerging Treatment Approaches and Future Directions

This section addresses emerging treatment approaches and future directions in Lyme disease management. It discusses ongoing research and developments in areas such as novel antibiotics, immunotherapies, and targeted therapies. The chapter explores potential advances in treatment options, including the development of vaccines against Borrelia burgdorferi and co-infections.

The section also highlights the importance of research on improved diagnostic tools to aid in early detection and timely treatment. It explores the potential benefits of point-of-care testing or more sensitive and specific serological assays to facilitate prompt diagnosis and appropriate treatment initiation.

Furthermore, the chapter discusses the significance of continued research and collaboration among scientists, clinicians, and patients to further understand the complexities of Lyme disease and develop more effective treatment approaches. It emphasizes the need for clinical trials, data collection, and evidence-based guidelines to guide treatment decisions and optimize patient outcomes.

By providing a more thorough elaboration of Chapter 5, readers gain a deeper understanding of the treatment approaches for Lyme disease. This knowledge allows them to comprehend the rationale behind antibiotic therapy, the management strategies or persistent or chronic symptoms, and the potential future advancements in treatment options. It also highlights the need for individualized care and ongoing research to improve outcomes for individuals affected by Lyme disease.

**Lyme disease treatment**

*Antibiotics*
The three first -line oral antibiotics for Lyme disease include doxycycline , amoxicillin and Cefuroxime.

Ceftriaxone (Rocephin) administered intravenously is the preferred antibiotics for neurologic Lyme disease in the United States. For early Lyme disease , a short course of oral antibiotics can cure the majority of cases.

The use of antibiotics is essential for treating Lyme disease.

Without antibiotics treatment, the Lymes disease bacteria can evade the host immunity system, disseminate through the bloodstream, and persist in the body.

The antibiotics go into the bacteria and stop the multiplication of the bacteria or disrupt the cell wall of the bacteria and kill the bacteria.

The adverse effect of Lyme disease medications
The antibiotics can cause skin rashes, and if an itchy red rash develops, see your physician. Sometimes the symptoms worsens for the first few days on antibiotics.

This is called a Herxheimer reaction and occurs when the antibiotics start to kill the bacteria. In the first 24 to 48 hours, dead bacterial products stimulate the immune system to release inflammatory chemokines that can cause fever and achiness.

The most common side effects of the penicillin antibiotic is diarrhea and occasionally even serious cases caused by the bacteria Clostridium difficile. This bacterial overgrowth occurs due to antibiotics killing the good bacteria in our gut. Taking probiotics can help restore the good bacteria.

**Chapter 6**: Lyme Disease Co-Infections: Beyond Borrelia

6.1 Co-Infections Associated with Lyme Disease

This section focuses on the co-infections often associated with Lyme disease, which are caused by other tick-borne pathogens. It explores the prevalence of these co-infections in areas where Lyme disease is endemic and highlights the importance of considering them in individuals with suspected or confirmed Lyme disease.

The chapter discusses common co-infections, including Babesia, Anaplasma, and Bartonella. It explains the transmission dynamics of these pathogens, their clinical manifestations, and the potential overlap in symptoms with Lyme disease.

The section emphasizes that co-infections can complicate the diagnosis and management of Lyme disease, as they may require specific diagnostic tests and targeted treatment approaches.

## 6.2 Diagnostic Considerations for Co-Infections

This section addresses the diagnostic considerations for co-infections associated with Lyme disease. It discusses the challenges involved in diagnosing these co-infections, as they may present with similar symptoms to Lyme disease or other common illnesses.

The chapter emphasizes the importance of considering co-infections in individuals with atypical or severe manifestations, treatment failures, or persistent symptoms despite appropriate Lyme disease treatment.

Furthermore, the section explores the diagnostic methods available for co-infections, such as serological tests, PCR testing, and clinical assessments. It discusses the need for comprehensive testing that includes screening for various tick-borne pathogens to ensure accurate diagnosis and appropriate treatment.

## 6.3 Treatment Approaches for Co-Infections

This section delves into the treatment approaches for co-infections associated with Lyme disease. It discusses the commonly used antibiotics and treatment regimens for specific co-infections, such as Babesiosis, Anaplasmosis, and Bartonellosis.

The chapter emphasizes the importance of early detection and prompt treatment to minimize the complications associated with co-infections.

The section also explores the potential challenges in treating co-infections, such as antibiotic resistance or the need for combination therapy.

It discusses the importance of tailoring treatment plans based on the specific co-infection, the individual's medical history, and any potential drug interactions or contraindications.

## 6.4 Co-Infections and Treatment Outcomes

This section addresses the impact of co-infections on treatment outcomes in Lyme disease.

It discusses how the presence of co-infections can influence the course of illness, the response to treatment, and the duration of recovery.

The chapter explores the potential challenges in managing co-infections and the implications for long-term prognosis.

Furthermore, the section emphasizes the importance of comprehensive and individualized care for individuals with Lyme disease and co-infections.

It discusses the need for multidisciplinary approaches, involving infectious disease specialists, rheumatologists, and other relevant healthcare professionals, to address the complex nature of co-infections.

## 6.5 Prevention and Awareness of Co-Infections

This section focuses on prevention strategies and raising awareness about the co-infections associated with Lyme disease.

It emphasizes the significance of tick bite prevention measures, such as using repellents, wearing protective clothing, and conducting regular tick checks.

The chapter highlights the need for education and public awareness campaigns to promote the recognition and understanding of co-infections among healthcare providers and the general public.

Additionally, the section addresses the importance of timely diagnosis and appropriate treatment of co-infections.

It discusses the need for improved diagnostic tools and guidelines that incorporate screening for co-infections in individuals with suspected or confirmed Lyme disease.

By providing a more thorough elaboration of Chapter 6, readers gain a deeper understanding of the co-infections associated with Lyme disease.

This knowledge allows them to recognize the importance of considering co-infections in the diagnostic and treatment process, understand the challenges involved, and appreciate the need for prevention strategies and increased awareness about these additional tick-borne pathogens.

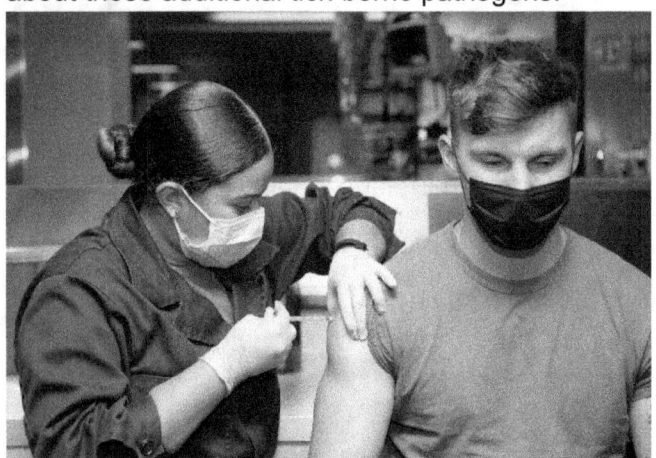

## Lyme disease and Co-infections

Tick-borne infections are zoonotic-

Zoonotic means they are passed from animals to humans.

"Vectors" like ticks , mosquitos and fleas transmit the diseases from animals like mice, rats, and squirrels to humans when they bite.

Ticks can carry many bacteria, viruses , fungi and protozoans all at the same time and transmit them in a single bite.

The most common tick-borne diseases in the United States include Lyme disease, babesiosis, anaplasmosis, ehrlichiosis, relapsing fever, tularemia, Rocky Mountain spotted fever (RMSF).

Diseases acquired together like this are called co-infections.

A person with a co-infection generally experiences more severe illness, more symptoms and a longer recovery.

**sporozoites** transferred during feeding

**multinucleated sporoblast**

sporozoites invade erythrocytes

kinetes invade the salivary glands

**binary fission** asexual reproduction

**kinete**

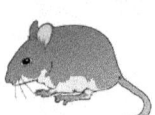

**deer tick** *Ixodes scapularis*

**white-footed mouse** *Peromyscus leucopus*

**merozoites**

**zygote** sexual reproduction

**ray bodies** Strahlenkörper

transferred to gut during feeding

infect additional erythrocytes

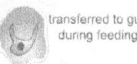

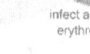

**gametogenesis**

**gametocytes**

## Babesia

Babesia is a malaria-like parasite that infects red blood cells. In addition to transmission by a tick, babesia can be transmitted from mother to unborn child or through a contaminated blood transfusion. Currently most blood banks do not screen donated blood for babesia.

## Symptoms of Babesiosis

The symptoms are similar to those of Lyme disease but more often starts with a high fever and chills. As the infection progresses, patients may develop fatigue, headaches , sweats, muscle spasms, chest pain, hip pain and shortness of breath.
 Babesiosis is often so mild it is not noticed but can be life-threatening to the elderly, to people with no spleen and people with a weak immune system.

Complications include very low blood pressure, severe hemolytic anemia (a breakdown of red blood cells and kidney failure.

Babesiosis is typically treated with a combination of ant-malarial drugs and antibiotics. Relapses sometimes occur after treatment and must be retreated.

## Bartonella

Bartonella are bacteria that live primarily inside the lining of the blood vessels. They can infect humans, mammals and a wide range of wild animals. The disease that results is called bartonellosis. It is mainly carried by cats and causes cat-scratch disease, endocarditis, and several other serious diseases in humans.

### Transmission of Bartonella

Bartonella bacteria are known to be carried by fleas, body lice and ticks, and there's high suspicion that ticks transmit it to humans. People with tick bites and no known exposure to cats have acquired the disease.

### Symptoms of Bartonellosis

Early signs include fever, fatigue , headaches , poor appetite  and an unusual streaked rash that resembles " stretch marks". Swollen glands are typical.  Neurological symptoms include blurred vision, numbness in the extremities, memory loss, balance problems, headaches, ataxia (unsteady gait), and tremors.

Treatment of Bartonellosis_ Fluoroquinolones and doxycycline are sometimes successful in treating it. However, some doctors report the need to use several antibiotics in combination.

## Rickettsia- Rocky Mountain Spotted Fever

(RMSF) is the most common rickettsial infection in the U.S. it can range from mild illness to a fatal one.

## Symptoms of RMSF

Initial symptoms include severe headaches, high fever, abdominal pain and muscle pain. It often-though not always - includes a spotted rash that begins at the wrist and/or ankles , and spreads outwards from there. The progression of RMSF varies greatly between patients. Some may recover quickly on oral medications , while others may require intravenous antibiotics, prolonged hospitalization or intensive care.

RMSF weakens small blood vessels throughout the body, giving rise to its characteristic rash. This widespread damage to the blood vessels allows the bacteria to spread to the heart and brain- and can quickly lead to death in those under age 4,m over age 60, or those whose immune systems are compromised.

Prior to the use of antibiotics, Rocky mountain Spotted fever had a fatality rate of 80%. In the U.S today, the fatality rate is 5%-10%.

## Ehrlichia and Anaplasma- Ehrlichiosis

Ehrlichia and Anaplasma is a term that describes several different bacterial diseases, one of which is also called anaplasmosis. Some are transmitted by tIxodes ticks and others by the lone star tick.
Symptoms

The clinical manifestation of ehrlichiosis and anaplasmosis are the same. It includes high fever, fatigue, muscle aches, and headaches. The disease can be mild or life-threatening. Severely ill patients can have a low blood white blood count, low platelet count, anemia, elevated liver enzymes, kidney failure and respiratory insufficiency. Older people or people with immune suppression are more likely to require hospitalization. Death has occurred.

## Treatment
The treatment of choice for ehrlichiosis and anaplasmosis is doxycycline, with rifampin. In resistant or complicated cases, combination antibiotic therapy may be  necessary to eradicate the                                                        infection.

**Chapter 7:** Prevention and Control Strategies: Promoting Tick Bite Prevention

7.1 Understanding Tick Behavior and Habitat

This section focuses on understanding tick behavior and habitat to develop effective prevention and control strategies. It explores the life cycle, feeding habits, and preferred habitats of tick vectors, such as black-legged ticks (Ixodes scapularis and Ixodes pacificus) in North America.

The chapter discusses how ticks thrive in wooded areas, tall grasses, and leaf litter, as well as their ability to survive in various climatic conditions.

Furthermore, the section highlights the importance of understanding tick seasonality and activity patterns. It discusses peak tick activity periods, typically during warmer months, and the need for heightened vigilance during these times.

The chapter emphasizes the significance of recognizing high-risk areas and tailoring prevention efforts                                  accordingly.

## 7.2 Personal Protection Strategies

This section provides practical information on personal protection strategies to prevent tick bites. It explores the use of protective clothing, such as long-sleeved shirts, long pants, and closed-toe shoes, to minimize exposed skin.

The chapter discusses the application of insect repellents containing DEET, picaridin, or permethrin on clothing and exposed skin surfaces to repel ticks.

Furthermore, the section delves into the importance of conducting regular tick checks
.
It provides guidance on performing thorough tick checks after potential exposure to tick-infested areas and discusses the proper techniques for safely removing attached ticks.

The chapter emphasizes the significance of early tick removal to reduce the risk of Lyme disease transmission.

## 7.3 Environmental Modifications and Tick Control

This section addresses environmental modifications and tick control measures to reduce tick populations and minimize human-tick encounters.

It discusses the importance of landscape management practices, such as keeping lawns mowed, removing leaf litter, and creating a physical barrier between wooded areas and living spaces.

The chapter explores the potential benefits of targeted acaricide (tick-control) treatments, especially in high-risk areas.

Additionally, the section explores the use of integrated pest management (IPM) approaches.

It discusses the combination of various strategies, including environmental modifications, targeted acaricide treatments, and the promotion of natural tick predators, to reduce tick populations and their impact on human health.

The chapter highlights the need for community engagement and cooperation to implement effective tick control measures.

## 7.4 Public Education and Awareness

This section addresses the importance of public education and awareness in preventing tick bites and reducing Lyme disease risk.

It discusses the need for comprehensive education campaigns targeting both the general public and high-risk groups, such as outdoor enthusiasts, hikers, and individuals residing in endemic areas.

The chapter explores the dissemination of accurate information about tick biology, disease transmission, and prevention strategies through various channels, including public health campaigns, educational materials, and online resources.

It emphasizes the significance of promoting awareness about the signs and symptoms of Lyme disease, the importance of early detection, and the appropriate actions to take in case of a tick bite.

## 7.5 Future Directions and Research

This section addresses future directions and research needs in tick bite prevention and control strategies. It discusses ongoing research efforts to develop new approaches, such as the development of novel acaricides, tick vaccines, or biological control methods targeting ticks and tick-borne pathogens.

The chapter also emphasizes the need for continued research to better understand tick behavior, habitat preferences, and the effectiveness of prevention strategies. It highlights the importance of collaborative efforts between researchers, public health agencies, and community stakeholders to address the challenges posed by ticks and Lyme disease effectively.

By providing a more thorough elaboration of Chapter 7, readers gain a deeper understanding of the prevention and control strategies for tick bites and Lyme disease. This knowledge allows them to implement effective personal protection measures, understand the significance of environmental modifications and tick control efforts, appreciate the importance of public education and awareness, and recognize the need for ongoing research to improve prevention strategies and reduce the burden of Lyme disease.

## How to remove a tick

Use clean , fine tipped tweezers to grasp the tick as close to the skin's surface as possible.

Pull upward with steady , even pressure. Don't twist or jerk the tick: this can cause the mouth -parts to break off and remain in the skin. If this happens, remove the mouth-piece easily with tweezers, leave it alone and let the skin heal.

After removing the tick, thoroughly clean the bit area and your hands with rubbing alcohol or soap and water.

Never crush a tick with your fingers. Dispose of a live tick by putting in alcohol, or a sealed bag, container or flushing it down the toilet.

## Follow-Up

If you develop a rash within several weeks of removing the tick, see your doctor.
. Tell the doctor about your recent tick bite.
. When the bit occurred, and where you most likely acquired                    the                    tick.

**Chapter 8**: Emotional and Psychological Impact

This section focuses on the emotional and psychological impact of living with Lyme disease. It explores the challenges and adjustments individuals face as they navigate the complexities of the disease and its impact on their daily lives.

The chapter discusses the emotional toll of dealing with chronic symptoms, uncertainty, and the potential for disrupted personal and professional lives.

Furthermore, the section addresses the psychological impact, such as anxiety, depression, and feelings of isolation, that can accompany a Lyme disease diagnosis.

It emphasizes the importance of recognizing and addressing these emotional and psychological challenges, both for individuals with Lyme disease and their loved ones.

## 8.2 Patient Support and Advocacy

This section delves into the importance of patient support and advocacy for individuals with Lyme disease. It explores the role of support groups, patient advocacy organizations, and online communities in providing a sense of belonging, understanding, and support.

The chapter discusses how these networks can help individuals cope with the challenges of Lyme disease by sharing experiences, exchanging information, and offering emotional support.

Additionally, the section emphasizes the significance of healthcare providers in offering compassionate care, listening to patients' concerns, and providing appropriate resources and referrals.

It explores the value of a collaborative approach between patients and healthcare professionals in managing the physical, emotional, and social aspects of living with Lyme disease.

## 8.3 Lifestyle Adjustments and Self-Care

This section addresses the lifestyle adjustments and self-care practices that individuals with Lyme disease can adopt to manage their condition.

It discusses the importance of developing a balanced lifestyle that includes adequate rest, nutrition, exercise, and stress management.

The chapter explores how these practices can contribute to overall well-being and symptom management.

Furthermore, the section explores the potential benefits of complementary and alternative therapies in supporting the management of Lyme disease symptoms.

It discusses practices such as acupuncture, herbal medicine, mindfulness, and yoga, highlighting the need for individualized approaches and consultation with healthcare professionals.

## 8.4 Communicating with Healthcare Providers

This section focuses on effective communication between individuals with Lyme disease and their healthcare providers.

It discusses the importance of open and honest dialogue, sharing symptoms and concerns, and actively participating in the decision-making process.

The chapter emphasizes the need for clear communication regarding treatment goals, expectations, and any challenges or side effects experienced.

Additionally, the section explores the importance of staying informed about the latest research and treatment options, and asking questions to clarify any uncertainties. It highlights the significance of building a collaborative relationship with healthcare providers to ensure comprehensive and personalized care.

8.5 Future Directions and Hope

This section addresses future directions and provides a message of hope for individuals living with Lyme disease. It discusses ongoing research efforts aimed at improving diagnostic tools, treatment options, and preventive measures. The chapter emphasizes the importance of staying informed about advancements in the field and being proactive in accessing appropriate care.

Furthermore, the section explores the resilience and strength demonstrated by individuals living with Lyme disease. It emphasizes the potential for managing symptoms, finding effective treatment approaches, and leading fulfilling lives. The chapter encourages individuals to remain hopeful and seek support from healthcare providers, support networks, and community resources.

By providing a more thorough elaboration of Chapter 8, readers gain a deeper understanding of the emotional and psychological impact of Lyme disease, the importance of patient support and advocacy, the value of lifestyle adjustments and self-care practices, effective communication with healthcare providers, and a sense of hope for the future.

This knowledge allows individuals with Lyme disease to navigate their journey with resilience, seek appropriate support, and take an active role in their overall well-being.

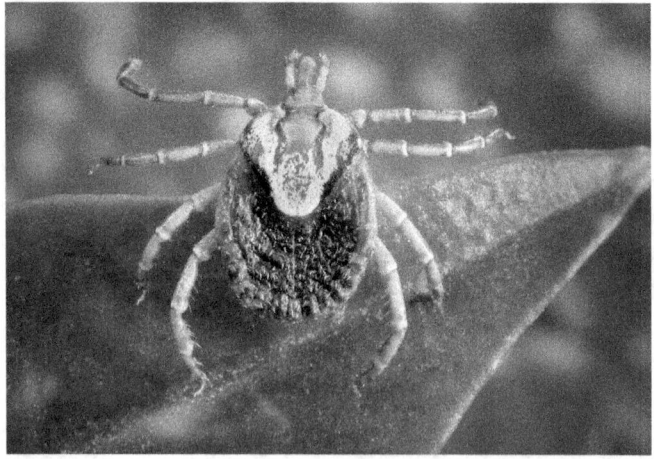

## Lyme Disease and Exercise

Lyme disease can have varying effects on individuals, and its impact on exercise and physical activity may differ from person to person. It's essential to consider the stage of the disease, the severity of symptoms, and individual health factors before engaging in any exercise routine. Here's a general overview of how Lyme disease can relate to exercise:

### Rest During Acute Phase:

In the acute phase of Lyme disease, when symptoms are most severe, it's crucial to prioritize rest and allow the body to recover. Symptoms during this stage may include fever, fatigue, muscle and joint pain, and headaches.

Engaging in strenuous exercise during this time can exacerbate symptoms and hinder the body's healing process.

Gradual Return to Exercise:

As the acute symptoms subside and antibiotic treatment progresses, individuals may gradually reintroduce light exercise or physical activity. Start with gentle activities such as walking or stretching to avoid overexertion.

**Listen to Your Body**: Pay close attention to how your body responds to exercise. If you experience increased fatigue, pain, or other symptoms, it's crucial to scale back and allow more time for recovery.

Remember that every individual's experience with Lyme disease can be different, and some may recover more quickly than others. Always prioritize your health and well-being and consult with a healthcare professional to determine the most appropriate exercise plan based on your current health status and symptoms.

**Manage Joint Pain and Inflammation:**

Lyme disease can sometimes lead to joint inflammation and pain. Low-impact exercises like swimming or biking may be more comfortable and less stressful on the joints.

**Avoid Overexertion**: Lyme disease can cause persistent fatigue, even after treatment. Avoid pushing yourself too hard, and remember that rest is an essential part of the recovery process.

**Seek Professional Guidance**: If you've been diagnosed with Lyme disease or suspect you may have it, consult with a healthcare professional before starting or resuming any exercise regimen. They can provide personalized advice based on your specific health condition.

**Preventive Measures**: If you are in an area with a high risk of tick exposure, consider taking preventive measures, such as wearing protective clothing, using insect repellent, and checking for ticks after spending time outdoors. Preventing Lyme disease is always better than treating it.

Lyme disease can negatively affect relationships, finances, cognition, emotions and quality of life and all aspects of daily functioning.

The researchers have found  that people with Lyme disease has a greater risk of mental problems and suicide  attempts. They also found they found that they had a 42% higher incident of depression and bipolar disorder, and a 75% higher risk of death by suicide,  compare  with  people  without  Lyme disease.

In severe cases, people with late stage Lyme disease may experience poor concentration, memory  and sleep disorders.

The longer that Lyme disease goes untreated, the more likely a patient is to develop these symptoms and disorders.

Talk to those close to you about the way that Lyme disease affects you. You and your loved ones can benefit from joining a support group for people with Lyme                                        disease.

**Chapter 9**: Lyme Disease Research and Future Perspectives

9.1 Importance of Research in Lyme Disease

This section focuses on the importance of research in advancing our understanding of Lyme disease. It discusses how research plays a crucial role in unraveling the complexities of the disease, improving diagnostic tools, developing more effective treatments, and enhancing prevention strategies. The chapter emphasizes that research is essential for addressing knowledge gaps, improving patient outcomes, and reducing the global burden of Lyme disease.

9.2 Current Research Areas

This section explores the current research areas in Lyme disease. It discusses ongoing studies and investigations aimed at improving diagnostic methods, understanding the pathogenesis of the disease, and optimizing treatment approaches. The chapter may delve into research on tick behavior and habitats, the genetic diversity of Borrelia burgdorferi strains, and the development of vaccines or novel therapeutics.

Furthermore, the section addresses research efforts to understand the long-term outcomes and potential complications associated with Lyme disease.
It may explore studies on the impact of co-infections, the persistence of symptoms after treatment, and the underlying mechanisms of chronic Lyme disease.

The chapter discusses the significance of these research endeavors in improving patient care and informing clinical practice.

9.3 Emerging Technologies and Innovations

This section addresses emerging technologies and innovations in Lyme disease research.

It discusses the potential of novel diagnostic tools, such as point-of-care tests or multiplex assays capable of detecting multiple tick-borne pathogens simultaneously.

The chapter explores advancements in imaging techniques, such as magnetic resonance imaging (MRI) or positron emission tomography (PET), for visualizing the effects of Lyme disease on various body systems.

Additionally, the section delves into the use of genomics, proteomics, and other "-omics" technologies to gain a deeper understanding of Borrelia burgdorferi and host interactions.

It discusses how these technologies can provide insights into the pathogenesis of Lyme disease, identify biomarkers for diagnosis or treatment response, and guide personalized treatment approaches.

## 9.4 Future Directions and Challenges

This section addresses future directions and challenges in Lyme disease research. It discusses the need for continued research efforts to improve diagnostic accuracy, especially in early stages of the disease, and enhance treatment outcomes.

The chapter emphasizes the significance of collaboration among researchers, clinicians, and public health agencies to address the challenges posed by Lyme disease effectively.

Furthermore, the section explores the importance of translational research that bridges the gap between laboratory findings and clinical practice.

It highlights the need for evidence-based guidelines, standardized treatment protocols, and improved dissemination of research findings to inform healthcare providers and optimize patient care.

## 9.5 Global Perspective and Public Health Implications

This section addresses the global perspective and public health implications of Lyme disease research.
It discusses the varying prevalence of Lyme disease worldwide and the need for research efforts in areas beyond traditional endemic regions.

The chapter emphasizes the importance of a global approach to understanding the disease, improving surveillance systems, and implementing preventive measures.

Additionally, the section explores the impact of climate change on tick distribution and disease transmission patterns.

It discusses the potential implications for public health and the importance of research in developing adaptive strategies to address these challenges.

By providing a more thorough elaboration of Chapter 9, readers gain a deeper understanding of the importance of research in Lyme disease, the current research areas and emerging technologies, future directions and challenges, and the global perspective and public health implications of Lyme disease research.

This knowledge enables individuals involved in research, healthcare providers, and policymakers to appreciate the significance of ongoing research efforts and work towards improving diagnosis, treatment, and prevention strategies for Lyme disease.

## The Lyme Disease Vaccine

Pfizer (US) and Valneva (Paris) Institute Initiate Phase 3 Study of Lyme Disease vaccine VLA15.

This is the only vaccine for Lyme disease in development. This vaccine will target the outer surface protein A (OspA) of Borrelia burgdorferi. The OspA is surface protein expressed by the bacteria when present in a tick. Blocking OspA inhibits the bacteria to leave the tick and infect humans.

The vaccine covers the 6 most common osspA serotypes expressed by the Borreliaburgdorferisensu lato species that are prevalent in North America and Europe.

The vaccine has shown a strong immune response and satisfactory profile in pre-clinical and clinical studies so far.

Valneva and Pfizer entered into a collaboration agreement in April 2020 to co-develop VLA15.

## History of a Failed Lyme Vaccine

25 years ago, a vaccine called LYMErix was created by Smithklinebeeham that was shown to be 76% effective at preventing Lyme disease.

However, by 2002, the vaccine was pulled by the pharmaceutical company due to poor sales.

The company also faced a class action lawsuit alleging that LyMerix caused arthritis in vaccinated individuals.

The FDA investigation concluded that the vaccine was not the cause, but by that time the demand for the vaccine had already plummeted.

Global Warming and infectious diseases.

The number of Lymes disease cases reported to the Center for Disease Control and Prevention has more than doubled in the last 20 years.

More than 475,000 people are diagnosed or treated for Lyme disease each year. Once contained to a small section of Northeast U.S and Midwest, Lyme disease cases have skyrocketed in those regions, and tick borne diseases are proliferating in Western states.

The dogs have been vaccinated against Lyme disease for more than 30 years but there is no present vaccination against Lyme disease in humans as of yet.

Famous People with Lyme Disease

. Avril Lavigne

. Alec Baldwin

. Bella Hadid

. Justin Biever

. Ben Stiller

. Kelly Osbourne

. Shaina Twain

. Amy Schumer

. Debbie Gibson

. Kris Kristofferson

. Mark Ruffalo

. Ryan Sutter

**Chapter 10**: The Global Impact of Lyme Disease

10.1 Global Distribution and Prevalence

This section focuses on the global distribution and prevalence of Lyme disease. It discusses how Lyme disease is no longer limited to specific regions and has become a global health concern. The chapter explores the varying prevalence of the disease in different parts of the world, including endemic areas in North America, Europe, Asia, and Australia.

Furthermore, the section addresses the factors contributing to the global spread of Lyme disease. It discusses the influence of changing climate patterns, deforestation, increased human mobility, and the expansion of tick populations and their habitats. The chapter emphasizes the need for global collaboration and surveillance to monitor the spread and impact of Lyme disease.

Additionally, the section explores the public health implications of Lyme disease. It discusses the challenges in accurately diagnosing and reporting cases, which can affect disease surveillance and control efforts.

The chapter emphasizes the need for standardized diagnostic protocols, improved reporting systems, and enhanced awareness among healthcare providers and the general public to mitigate the impact of Lyme disease on public health.

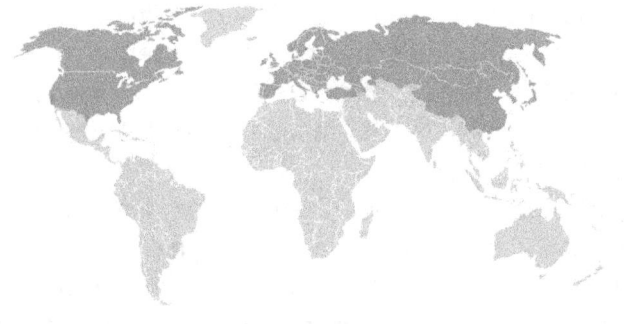

## 10.2 Challenges in Diagnosis and Treatment

This section addresses the challenges in diagnosing and treating Lyme disease on a global scale. It discusses the limitations of diagnostic tests, particularly in regions where the disease is emerging or where co-infections are prevalent.

The chapter explores the need for research and development of improved diagnostic tools that can detect various Borrelia burgdorferi strains and co-infections accurately.

Furthermore, the section explores the challenges in treatment, including variations in clinical presentation, treatment response, and availability of healthcare resources.
It discusses the importance of raising awareness among healthcare providers in regions with emerging Lyme disease cases and ensuring access to appropriate treatment options.

The chapter emphasizes the need for global guidelines and treatment recommendations that consider regional variations and address the challenges faced by healthcare systems worldwide.

## 10.3 Prevention Strategies and Awareness

This section focuses on prevention strategies and raising awareness about Lyme disease on a global scale. It discusses the importance of educating the public about the risks of tick bites, the recognition of early symptoms, and the adoption of personal protection measures.

The chapter explores the role of public health campaigns, educational programs, and community engagement in promoting tick bite prevention and early detection of Lyme disease worldwide.

Additionally, the section addresses the need for international collaboration in sharing best practices, research findings, and prevention strategies. It discusses the importance of knowledge exchange among countries to address the global impact of Lyme disease collectively.

The chapter emphasizes the significance of fostering partnerships between researchers, healthcare providers, policymakers, and public health agencies to develop effective prevention and control                                        programs.

## 10.5 Future Directions and Global Cooperation

This section addresses future directions and the importance of global cooperation in addressing the impact of Lyme disease. It discusses the need for continued research to improve diagnostic accuracy, treatment outcomes, and preventive measures.

The chapter explores the potential for global collaboration in sharing data, research findings, and best practices to enhance disease surveillance, control efforts, and patient care.

Furthermore, the section emphasizes the significance of interdisciplinary approaches and collaboration between scientists, clinicians, policymakers, and community stakeholders.

It discusses the importance of integrating knowledge from various fields, such as epidemiology, entomology, immunology, and climate science, to understand the complex dynamics of Lyme disease globally.

By providing a more thorough elaboration of Chapter 10, readers gain a deeper understanding of the global impact of Lyme disease. This knowledge enables individuals involved in public health, research, healthcare provision, and policymaking to appreciate the extent of the disease worldwide, address the challenges in diagnosis and treatment, implement effective prevention strategies, and work towards global cooperation to mitigate the impact of Lyme disease on a global scale.

## Lyme disease and Health cost

An estimated 240,000 to 440,000 people are diagnosed with Lyme disease each year, with an average of 3,000 spent annually per patient on treatment according to one study, published in PLOS ONE. Treating Lyme disease can cost the health care system up to 1.3 billion annually. The effective prevention and early diagnosis of Lyme disease are important to reduce illness and associated                                    cost.

The interdisciplinary approach in Lyme disease

. Epidemiology- The branch of medicine which deals with the incident, distribution and possible control of diseases and other factors relating to health.
. Entomology-The branch of zoology (animal) that concerns the study of insects.
. Immunology- Is the study of the immune system.
. Rheumatologist- Is a specialist who diagnoses and treats arthritis and other immune-related diseases and conditions.
. Cardiologist- Is a physician who is an expert in the care of the heart and blood vessels.
. Neurologist- A doctor who treats nervous system disorders.
. Infectious disease doctor- A doctor who specializes in the diagnosis and treatment of complex infections. They can also treat people with long-term (chronic) infections or disorders.

## Homeopathic Nosodes approach

Nosodes are highly diluted noxious substances that elicit the body's natural immune response. The homeopathic nosodes alert the immune system to go after the specific pathogen and co-infections.
The specific herbs (nosodes) which may include lemon balm, Sarsaparila and cat's claws.

Nutritional products contain ingredients such as fulvic acid , probiotics and activated charcoal which mop up the released toxins while protecting your organs and system from any damage.
Follow a healthy maintenance routine like a healthy diet, exercise, good hydration and stress management to keep your immune system strong and prevent future infections.

## Essential Oil for Lyme disease

It's believed that many essential oils have antimicrobial activities. Researchers have tested 34 essential oils against the bacteria that causes Lyme disease (not in humans) and found that cinnamon, clove bud, citronella, wintergreen and oregano show strong activity against the bacterium. Even more effective than daptomycin, the "gold standard " antibiotic many people with Lyme disease prescribed.

**Other treatments includes:**

. Acupuncture

. Bee venom

. Stem cell transplantation

. Sauna

. Stevia

. Chelation Therapy

. Magnet

. Nutrition Therapy

. Enemas

## Support Groups for Lyme Disease

- Lyme Disease.org
- Global Lyme Alliance
- Lyme Connection
- Generation Lyme
- Lyme Light Foundation
- Lyme Disease Association
- National Capital Lyme
- Facebook: Women's Lyme disease
- Lyme Basics. Org
- Project Lyme.org
- Lymelaser.com
- Lyme Warrior

Lyme disease is a complex and multisystemic illness caused by the bacteria Borrelia burgdorferi and transmitted through the bite of infected ticks. It poses a significant public health challenge globally, with varying prevalence and distribution in different regions
The disease progresses through different stages, with distinct signs and symptoms. Early diagnosis and prompt treatment are essential to prevent complications and long-term health effects.

The diagnosis of Lyme disease can be challenging due to the nonspecific nature of symptoms and limitations of available diagnostic tests. Healthcare providers must consider clinical evaluation, medical history, and potential exposure to infected ticks to make an accurate diagnosis.
 Ongoing research aims to improve diagnostic tools and guidelines, ensuring early detection and appropriate treatment.
Antibiotic therapy is the primary treatment approach for Lyme disease. Timely and adequate treatment can effectively control the infection and prevent complications. However, some individuals may experience persistent or chronic symptoms despite treatment, requiring comprehensive management and multidisciplinary care.

Prevention plays a crucial role in reducing the burden of Lyme disease. Personal protection measures, such as wearing protective clothing, Using insect repellents, and conducting regular tick checks, are essential for minimizing tick bites. Environmental modifications, tick control measures, and public education campaigns are crucial for preventing tick bites and raising awareness about the disease. Living with Lyme disease can have emotional, psychological, and socioeconomic impacts on individuals and their families. Patient support networks, advocacy organizations, and healthcare providers play a vital role in offering support, sharing information, and promoting self-care strategies. Ongoing research, global cooperation, and interdisciplinary approaches are essential for advancing our understanding of Lyme disease, improving diagnostics, treatment outcomes, and prevention strategies on a global scale.

In conclusion, Lyme disease is a complex illness that requires a comprehensive approach involving prevention, early diagnosis, appropriate treatment, and support for individuals living with the disease. By increasing awareness, promoting research, and fostering collaboration, we can better address the challenges posed by Lyme disease and work towards reducing its global impact on public health.

## References

Center for Disease Control and Prevention: Lyme Disease (2022). CDC. Retrieved from www.cdc.gov

Lyme Disease: Diagnosis and Treatment (2022). Mayo Clinic. Retrieved from www.mayoclinic.org

Medline Plus: Lyme Disease (2020). Medline Plus. Retrieved from www.medlineplus.gov

Lyme Disease: Symptoms, treatments, prevention and recovery (2022). Cleveland clinic. Retrieved from https://my.clevelandclinic.org

www.ingramcontent.com/pod-product-compliance
Lightning Source LLC
Chambersburg PA
CBHW062340290526
45794CB00005B/2062